WEIGHT LOSS SECRET

Aaron Blake

Disclaimer

The information contained in this book is designed to provide helpful information on the subjects discussed. This book is sold with the understanding that the authors and publisher are not engaged in rendering medical, health, or any other kind of personal professional services in the book. As with all exercise and dietary programs, you should consult your physician before beginning. The publisher and author specifically disclaim all responsibility for any liability, loss, or risk, personal or otherwise, which is incurred as a consequence, directly or indirectly, of the use and application of any of the contents of this book.

Table of Contents

Introduction

We do so well at achieving goals and with the things we want in life. However, a majority of us struggle with controlling our weight. It only becomes more difficult as times moves forward. As we progress through life we walk a tight rope trying to balance family, work, and our ever increasing responsibilities. To put the icing on the cake, information is flooding our senses making it difficult to know what to believe or what to do. Often times, information conflicts with other information. So what are we to do? Unfortunately, we either never figure it out or we learn the hard and painful way. I learned from the later.

My family was poor growing up. My mother divorced my father when I was very young. Being a single mother, she struggled to provide for us. I didn't have a lot of clothes and we couldn't afford to get them cleaned very often at the laundry mat. I was bullied for always wearing the same clothes and stinking. I remember going days without eating. When pay day came around, my mom always bought McDonalds for dinner until the money was gone. Then we went without food until the next pay check rolled in. Every Christmas I woke up to find a tree with no presents underneath it. I lived like this until I barely graduated high school. After graduation I joined the U.S. Air Force.

After joining the military I was finally able to afford a wardrobe. More importantly, I was finally able to eat three meals a day. I was never taught healthy eating habits and needless to say, I slowly began gaining weight. It didn't help that, because of my job which was a fighter aircraft mechanic, I didn't get a lunch break during my 12 hour shifts. I was so hungry when I got home that I gorged myself for dinner. Also, I wasn't granted gym time during my work hours (like the rest of the military was). We were expected to work out on our own. Foregoing the gym was easy after being tired and hungry from a long shift and from having a family commitment. It eventually took its toll and got to the point that my military career was threatened due to my lack of fitness. This didn't just happen to me, a large percentage of us in this career field struggled with this very same issue! I eventually reached a tipping point where my waist measured over 40 inches, which was an automatic failure on my fitness tests.

Because of failing my fitness test, I was automatically enrolled in the Air Force's Fitness Improvement Program (FIP), or better known as "fat boy class." I had to sit through classes and listen to overweight instructors telling me how to eat healthy. They obviously didn't practice what they preached. I finally got my gym time as part of my work day. Unfortunately, these fitness sessions were led by a random person who didn't have a clue what they were doing. In a desperate attempt to improve my fitness, I also went to the gym after work. I was going to the gym twice a day. Yet my waist circumference was not getting smaller and at times it was actually getting bigger!

The stress was unbearable! I felt hopeless. I didn't feel comfortable in my own skin. I felt trapped in my body. I felt like I let my family down, let my country down, and worse I let myself down. I had felt as if everyone was constantly judging me by the way they looked at me. I had read so many books. I tried different diets such as the Atkins diet. Typically, I dropped a few pounds, but that was it. The diets were unhealthy, extreme, and impossible to continue with for a long period of time. Eventually I gained the weight back and then some. I finally hit rock bottom when I was kicked out of the military for failing to maintain fitness standards.

It was only after my downfall that I finally learned how to lose weight. I'm sure you can relate to some of these struggles such as trouble finding time to exercise. I'm sure work and family obligations add complexity to the issue. The hardest part for me was overcoming my emotional eating. Because of my past and current struggles at the time, it was almost as if I couldn't control myself. I knew that I shouldn't eat a certain way and it didn't matter how much I fought, I still gave in and felt guilty afterwards. This was a horrible cycle to be trapped in and it was hard to break. I eventually figured out what to do and broke free. The good news is that you can too!

Why should you listen to me? I'm not an expert. I'm not naturally skinny. However, I'm also not some overweight person pulling the "do as I say, not as I do" card. The struggle is real. I've gone through it and survived. That is what qualifies me to write this book. I have experienced it firsthand. I understand what you're going through and what it takes to shed those seemingly impossible pounds.

In many of his books, Tony Robbins has said that having knowledge or information is useless if you don't use it. You can know everything there is to know about something, but it will mean nothing if you don't put that knowledge to use. Tony Robbins goes on to say that using your knowledge is mastery. I agree. And for this reason, this book is intended to be short. I'm not going to waste your time droning on with filler just to reach a high page count. This book will be candid and to the point. It will give you the necessary techniques, methods, tools, and knowledge for weight loss without belaboring the point. This book will be short to allow you to immediately begin using the information in order to gain mastery.

This book isn't for everyone. This book is not for individuals who are not serious about taking control of their weight. This book is not for those who want to join the latest fad diet. It is only meant for those who are truly ready to be in control. It is only meant for those who are ready to cut through the mass amounts of misinformation to learn the true secret to weight loss.

Together we will talk about some important aspects regarding this weight loss journey. You will learn the secret to losing weight. The secret has become buried in the overwhelming and contradicting information that we are inundated with. We will combine these aspects to build a plan which will be *your* strategy to lose weight. With this secret, you will immediately begin losing weight and your life will drastically start changing as you start receiving compliments within days of implementing your plan.

The method used to lose weight is actually very simple and is not convoluted or complex. You will immediately see results. Seeing the results coupled with the methods we cover will motivate you to continue and finally achieve the weight loss you always wanted! Are you excited? I am, because I know it works. Let's get started!

Get off the Bandwagon

While in high school I worked at Burger King. I always worked swing shift and closed the kitchen. I worked with the same manager just about every night. We'll call her Jean. Jean was a good manager and a good person. She was also very overweight. Just about every other week she would tell me how she was doing the latest fad diet. She also told me just about every other week how she had lost 20 pounds. However, she always looked the same to me. After I graduated high school, I quit and joined the Air Force. About a year after joining, I went back to my home town for Christmas vacation. I stopped in at Burger King to visit my old friends that still worked there. Jean was still working there and as usual told me how much weight she had lost. Once again, she still looked the same. Does this sound familiar? Jean isn't the only person I know that acts like this. I came name a few others right now!

Who can blame Jean? I've tried fad diets in the past. Often times I would lose the first five pounds quickly and then the weight loss stopped. I was always excited about the new diet and bragged about it to my friends. So when it stopped working, I lied. After all, nobody likes to admit they're wrong. I would eventually move on to the next latest fad diet and brag about that one to my friends too. After many botched attempts, I finally learned that fad diets don't work.

To be fair, I do know a handful of people who have tried these diets and did seem to lose weight. There was only one major problem. They couldn't sustain the diet. They eventually gained the weight back and more. I typically gained more weight back after my own botched attempts.

We all get caught up in the hype. Different diets such as Atkins, Paleo, or the latest Wheat Belly diet are so easy to get caught up in. They seem to make sense. They do such a good job with marketing that you see it on the book shelves in stores, on the news, in commercials, and even multiple friends talk about it. So we get wrapped up in the hype and jump on the diet bandwagon out of fear that we are missing out on something great.

I quickly learned through disappointing failures that completely eliminating one type of food does not work. The Atkins diet starts off this way. The Paleo diet, or better known as the Caveman diet, is another silly fad. History has shown us that hunter gathers such as caveman were mostly malnourished and died of starvation. So following something like the Paleo diet is complete nonsense to me. The more recent fad diet is the Wheat Belly diet. Almost overnight, two-thirds of the people I know all of the sudden had a "gluten allergy." This has become such a fad that I now seeing food products proudly displaying that they are "gluten free" on the label. Often times these foods never had gluten in them to begin with. People buy into these diets so completely that they automatically become offended and defensive when you disagree.

These diets will eventually be replaced by a new fad diet. They always are. Instead of jumping on the bandwagon, you are about to discover what really works. Before we move on I would like to say one more thing.

After telling my friends and family about starting diets they always had comments to make when I failed. Some people seemed to go out of their way to sabotage me or get in my head with negative comments. There are many people who are naysayers and want to see you fail. I would challenge you to keep your weight loss a secret. It is no one else's business. Also, it is so exciting when those around you begin asking, "Have you been losing weight?" It is extremely motivating and boosts your confidence. So have fun with it!

Emotionally Drive Human Beings

Humans are emotionally driven. Emotions such as fear, greed, happiness, sadness, and many others drive us. Two dominate emotions that drive us to take action are pain and pleasure. Generally speaking, we are either moving towards or away from these emotions.

There was a time when I had gotten into a bad habit of eating McDonalds for lunch every day. I knew that it wasn't healthy for me. I would even bring a lunch to work and still decide to go to McDonalds instead. But why? I knew McDonalds was unhealthy and I had good intentions by bringing a lunch; however, I kept making the poor choice. It was because I was being emotionally driven which always trumped my good intentions.

I realized that I had been getting very annoyed with my coworkers. We didn't have a break room so we ate our lunch in our cubicles. Going to McDonalds gave me an excuse to get out of the office so I could get alone time. Once I realized this, I decided to start walking on my lunch. This completely solved my problem. I was back to eating a healthy sensible lunch and getting alone time to help me tolerate those coworkers that annoyed me. There is a very important lesson behind this story.

These two emotions may be partially responsible for your weight. If you find comfort in food every time something bad or stressful happens, your desire to feel pleasure might be what drives you to eat more or to eat certain types of foods that may not be healthy. Pain and pleasure performs a tug of war on your actions for various reasons causing you to eat or behave in various different ways. When these two emotions work in tandem, it doesn't matter what our intentions are or how strong will we try to be, we become powerless and give in.

Often times our emotional responses are triggered by events or even objects. It is important for you to sit down and take the time to identify triggers that may cause you to make poor food choices. Think about where you eat and the kind of foods you eat throughout your week. Also, take note of the circumstances, events, time of day, or the people you're interacting with such as family, friends, or coworkers when making poor food choices. This will help you identify triggers. After thoughtful consideration and analysis, you should begin to see patters and obvious triggers emerge. You will then be able to find ways to adapt your responses or avoid these triggers all together.

Once you have identified the triggers, you can now decide on ways to avoid these triggers. I realized that a large part of my overeating stemmed from my childhood when I would go days without food. So when I did eat, I gorged myself because subconsciously I didn't know when I would get my next meal. I was able to fix this by keeping plenty of food in my house as reassurance. I eventually learned that I didn't need to eat as much at each sitting because there was plenty of food available. Identifying annoying coworkers as a trigger to go out to McDonalds every day for lunch helped me make healthy changes.

The possible triggers that elicit emotional responses are endless. It can be a simple as seeing your favorite fast food sign as you drive home from work. Perhaps a solution would be to drive a different route home and break the habit. Or perhaps you might find a trigger that will require you to avoid certain social situations or certain individuals all together.

To summarize, we are emotionally drive. Identify the triggers that cause you to emotionally react. Which for the purposes of this book, the reaction is typically unhealthy eating habits. Decide on ways to avoid these triggers or how you can alter the situation to help you make better eating habits. This strategy will go a long way towards the war we wage on being overweight. On a piece of paper, write down the triggers that you have identified. Now write how you will react in these situations. This will be an important part of your strategy.

SMART Goal

Not having a goal is similar to going for a road trip and not knowing where you're going, how to get there, or whether or not you have arrived. Done properly, a goal is an amazing motivational tool. Setting goals is the common denominator amongst influential and successful people. However, there are many people who do not know how to properly make goals. Entire books have been written on the subject. We're only going to touch the tip of the ice berg, but it will be sufficient for our purposes.

As with many areas of our lives, we will need to make goals to help challenge and motivate ourselves in our weight loss journey. Goals must be planned. They aren't something that you think about for five seconds and then forget. Also, goals should be written down. Your goals will become more real when put on paper. To help make goals, there is a four step planning process:

<u>Four-Step Basic Goal Planning Process</u>:

1. Situational awareness
2. Alternative goals
3. Goal planning
4. Implementation and evaluation

1. Situational Awareness

Situational awareness means becoming aware of your surroundings and the environment you find yourself in. This is where a problem is recognized. The problem is something that you have identified that needs to change. For example, the problem I became aware of was how unhappy I was about my weight.

2. Alternative Goals

Once you have identified an achievement, result, or some end-state that you want to achieve, you need to compile a list of goals that will help you achieve this end state. For instance I wanted to lose weight. Alternative goals might be to drink less soda.

Don't be critical when compiling your list. At this stage anything goes. The idea is just to get down every alternative goal that you can think of. After you have a list, move onto the next step.

3. Goal Planning

Take the list that you just compiled and evaluate each alternative. Which alternatives are better? Which alternatives are horrible? Start eliminating your list down to one long-term goal and some short-term goals that are in alignment with the long-term goal. It is time to develop your goal.

We often here goals like, "I want to lose weight." There's a high probability that you may have said this before. I certainly have. The above example is not a goal, it is a dream. What kind of weight is loss? A person can lose muscle, water, or fat. How much weight? When should this be accomplished by? A goal should be able to address these types of questions. That is exactly what a SMART goal does. A SMART goal is:

SMART:

Specific

Measurable

Attainable

Realistic

Time-bound

Specific

The goal needs to be specific. Sticking with the above example, our goal is to lose fat. Losing water and muscle is not what we are after here. Not to mention, it isn't healthy.

Measurable

Our goal must be measurable. We can weigh ourselves on a bathroom scale and measure whether or not we are successful in losing fat. If we can't measure our goal we won't know if we're going in the right direction and whether or not to change something.

Attainable

Our goal must be attainable. An attainable goal might be to lose eight pounds this month. Losing two pounds a week is considered a healthy amount of weight to lose in a week. Two pounds a week times four weeks in a month equals eight pounds a month. This is attainable. Expecting to lose a hundred pounds in one month is not attainable.

Realistic

Our goal must be realistic. If you weigh 200 pounds, wanting to lose 230 pounds would not be realistic. This example is extreme but it gets the point across. A goal should be challenging; however, it still needs to remain realistic. If it isn't realistic, we'll fail to reach our goal which will lead to frustration and eventually we would abandon all of our hard work. Finally, a goal must state when it needs to be accomplished by.

Time-Bound

A good goal is time-bound. This motivates people to work towards their goal. I think we can relate to the example of procrastination. People procrastinate until they have a dead-line to accomplish something. The pressure of this dead-line motivates people into action. The same is true with goals.

Completed SMART Goal

After following these steps you will have a SMART goal. So what does a properly stated goal look like?

Once again, here is my goal that was a failure. *I want to lose weight.*

Here is what this goal looks like properly stated as a SMART goal. *I want to lose eight pounds of fat by September 1ˢᵗ.* Let's evaluate the components of my SMART goal. I said I want to *lose fat*. This is specific. My goal says that I want to *lose eight pounds*. This is easily measureable with a bathroom scale. This goal is attainable because it is healthy to lose about two pounds of fat a week. There are four weeks in a month which equates to a healthy weight loss of eight pounds. This goal is realistic. Finally, this goal is time-bound. My goal is to lose this weight by *September 1ˢᵗ*. My new goal meets all of the requirements to be a SMART goal. It is specific, measurable, attainable, realistic, and it is time-bound.

When done properly, a SMART goal will motivate you. It also helps you determine if you're making progress. If not, than you may need to make some adjustments to what you are doing. Please take the time now to develop your own personal goal. You will be doing yourself a disservice by skipping this important step.

4. Implementation and Evaluation

Now that we have a goal we must implement it. After all, a decision doesn't do anybody any good if it is not acted upon. I was taught in the military that you have to make and implement a decision. Not acting is worse than making a bad decision. Just do something.

Once you have taken action and implemented your goal, you need to evaluate it. This is why a goal must be measurable, so that you can tell if it is working or not. Once again sticking with my weight loss goal, I will evaluate this goal by stepping on the bathroom scale to see if I'm losing two pounds a week. I can then make minor corrections to help achieve my goal. Perhaps I lost three pounds one week. I might need to adjust what I'm doing, such as consuming less calories, so I don't lose weight too quickly. Conversely, perhaps I only lost one pound and I need to make corrections so that I'm losing two.

Time to Believe

Never underestimate the power of the mind! Our state of mind can have a dramatic effect on the human body. The following is a perfect example.

Pretend that you are taking a small day trip. So you get in your car and drive out of town for a while to your favorite place for a small easy hike. After all, there's nothing better than a little nature therapy. You're walking on the dirt trail. You are surrounded by mountains and trees so tall you can barely see the sky. The shade is cool. Every now and again you feel an even cooler breeze because of the small creak that's not too far away. The wind dancing through the trees and the distant calming sound of water running relaxes you. All the sudden a bear runs onto the trail in front of you, stands on its hind legs growing two times taller than you, and letting out a deafening roar. Your heart jolts to a million beats per minute and your skin is covered in goose bumps as fear coerces through your veins.

The question is, did the bear cause your heart rate to jump and your skin to get goose bumps? If you answered no, you're absolutely right. The bear did not cause any of these things. How could it? It never physically touched you! Your mind is what causes these changes. The mind is so powerful that it has the capability of causing physiological changes to the body.

We can harness the power of our mind. There are things we can do to put ourselves in a resourceful state of mind. By putting ourselves in a resourceful state of mind, there is little that can stop us. I'm going to specifically talk about using affirmations. If you find this interesting and choose to research it further, there is an entire field dedicated to this. It is called Neuro Linguistic Programming (NLP). I think NLP is fascinating and the various techniques can be used to help us in so many different areas of our lives! But for now, we'll focus on using it to help with weight loss.

Develop Your Affirmation

You are probably familiar with affirmations. Some people repeat mantras such as, "I'm feeling good" or "I've got this!" You will be doing something a little different. You will be doing affirmations the way they were meant to be done and in a way that will be more effective. Your affirmation will help get you in a resourceful state of mind whenever you need it.

Start of by making a list of what you are hoping for as a result of your weight loss. This can be anything. The items you put on this list needs to have emotions tied behind it to be effective. For example, perhaps you want to be in better shape to be able to play with your children. It could be to look sexier for your spouse or the opposite sex.

Now that you have made your list, choose the one that you like most, the one with the most emotion, the one that motivates you.

This next step is very important. You need to visualize this in the first person. As if you are seeing it through your own eyes. Don't worry if you can't picture it perfectly with your eyes closed. The thought is enough. The more sensory information you can add to the visualization the better. For example, let's say you want to be able to play with your children. In this visualization you will be viewing it from your own eyes, see your children, here them laughing, see the green grass, smell the fresh air, and so on and so forth. Feel how great it is to be in better shape. If you develop your affirmation properly it will motivate you to make better choices. The point of the affirmation is to get you to experience the future state that you hope to be in. The human mind doesn't know the difference between reality and the visualization. By visualizing, you trick your mind into believing that you are already in that future state and this helps your mind to make the kinds of choices that would be required for you to be that way. To help better make my point, let me share with you the affirmation that I used.

I never considered myself to be very attractive to women. My affirmation was about me being skinny with a nice muscular physic. I would walk into different places such as the gym, a gas station, or a college class room and the women would stop what they were doing and check me out. I found my affirmation very motivating. It helped me be more confident and positive. More importantly, it motivated me to make the correct choice. When I was faced with a decision to eat healthy food or not, I took a minute to think about my affirmation which motivated me to choose healthy food because that's what it would take to have the kind of body that got women's attention. Sometimes I had the hard choice between exercising at the gym or just stay home. I took a few minutes to do my affirmation. It motivated me. I chose to go to the gym. This is the power of a well-developed affirmation!

Quiet before the Storm

Before moving forward, I think it is important to pause and reflect on what we have covered so far.

Most fad diets do not work. They can be extreme. They may completely remove specific foods from your diet. Often times, these banned foods contain nutrients that your body needs. Fad diets are hard to maintain which sets us up for failure. When certain types of diets are heavily marketed, restaurant chains jump on-board with providing the latest "miracle food," or food products in the supermarket that are proudly marked to support of a specific diet, then you know it is a fad diet and it would be in your best interest to steer clear. The fad diet will always become obsolete and be replaced by another. There's no need to follow the crowd and get caught up in the hype, because you will know the true secret to weight loss!

Our predominate emotions of pain and pleasure drive us to act. There are certain situations that trigger these emotions and therefore drive us to act. The actions we take, such as over eating or poor food choices, are partly responsible for the need to lose weight. By now you should have taken the time to identify the triggers that contribute to poor eating habits and identify ways to avoid or deal with these triggers. If not, please take the time now before moving forward.

Successful people set goals and you should too. More specifically, you should develop a SMART goal for weight loss. Just remember the SMART acronym to help. Your weight loss goal should be specific, measurable, attainable, realistic, and time-bound. Your SMART goal is a very powerful tool to motivate you, it provides feedback letting you know if your strategy is working or not, and will allow you to hold yourself accountable. If you didn't develop your goal during the chapter on SMART goals, then please stop and develop it now before moving forward.

It is now time to believe! The human mind is powerful. The mind is capable of eliciting physiological changes to the body. By harnessing this power, we can use our mind to willfully create changes in our lives. We will use affirmations to harness this power. We use affirmation by visualizing the end goal as if we have already achieved it. We will visualize in the first-person, through our own eyes. Exactly like how you experience your reality such as reading this book. The result of your weight loss should elicit a strong emotional response.

Our subconscious can't tell the difference between the past, present, or future. By picturing yourself already in this future state of having accomplished your weight loss, it will cause your subconscious to take actions which are in alignment with this new you. You should focus on your affirmation three times a day. Also, use your affirmation anytime when faced with a difficult decision such as choosing between a poor or a healthy food choice.

So far, everything that you have developed is part of your weight loss strategy. Your strategy consists of the knowledge that fad diets don't work and you don't need them anyways because you know the secret to weight loss. The secret that you are about to learn next. Your strategy will consist of knowing that you are emotionally driven, that you have identified your triggers, and have back-up plans for when these triggers occur. Your strategy contains your SMART goal and your affirmation. Now it is time to learn and add the weight loss secret to your plan.

The Magic Number

There are many articles, blogs, books, and experts who claim to show you how to lose weight and gain muscle at the same time. This is a myth. As a matter of fact, losing weight and gaining muscle at the same time is physiologically impossible! To gain muscle (or fat) you need a surplus of calories. To lose weight you need a deficit of calories. It is impossible to do both at the same time.

What is a Calorie?

We first need to understand what a calorie is. We have used this word and we have heard this word being used by others. For some of us it is something we talk about daily. But do we really understand exactly what it means?

A calorie is a unit of energy. More specifically, one calorie equals the amount of energy necessary to raise the temperature of one gram of water by one degree Celsius. Simply put, our bodies require energy to function. We receive this energy from the foods and drinks we consume. The amounts of energy contained in food and drinks we consume are measured in calories.

Basal Metabolic Rate

As mentioned previously, our bodies require energy to function. And here is the secret to weight loss that you have finally been waiting for! Our bodies require a very specific amount of energy to function. If our body receives the exact amount of energy it needs, we'll maintain our current weight. If we consume more calories than our body needs, it is stored as fat. If we consume fewer calories than our body needs, we will lose weight. The basal metabolic rate (BMR) is the amount of energy our body would need at rest. Another word, if we were to lie in bed for a 24 hour period and not move an inch, the basal metabolic rate is the minimum amount of energy that our body requires to function.

Most diets and food products base serving sizes on a "2,000 Calorie a day" diet. The problem with this is that every person is different. Not everyone will have the same rate of energy expenditure. As a matter of fact, the heavier a person is, the more calories they will need compared to a lighter person. The good news is we can calculate what our own BMR is. By knowing what our BMR is, we can begin to adjust the amount of calories we consume to lose weight. The BMR calculation for men and women are different. So feel free to jump to the section that explains how to calculate your BMR. Please don't feel intimidated by the math. I will walk you through the process of calculating your BMR.

Men Basal Metabolic Rate Calculation

First, let's use a hypothetical male as an example. His name will be Bill. In order for Bill to calculate his BMR he will need to know three pieces of information. Bill will need to know his weight in pounds, height in inches, and age in years.

Bill used his bathroom scale to determine that he weighs 270 pounds.

If you don't know your height, grab a friend and a tape measure. Bill knows that he is 5 foot 11. He needs to know his height in inches. To figure this out Bill will multiply 5 times 12, since there are 12 inches in a foot, the answer bill comes up with is 60. He then adds 11, since it is already in inches, to his previous answer of 60. Bill is 71 inches tall.

Finally, Bill knows that he is 30 years old.

Now that Bill has collected the three required pieces of information, we can finally begin to calculate Bill's BMR. The BMR calculation for men is:

$$BMR = 66 + (6.23 \times Weight\ in\ pounds)$$

$$+ (12.7 \times Height\ in\ inches)$$

$$- (6.8 \times Age\ in\ years)$$

First, write out the equation and substitute the required information with your weight, height, and age. Here is what the equation looks like with Bill's information:

$$BMR = 66 + (6.23 \times 270) + (12.7 \times 71) - (6.8 \times 30)$$

Following the order of operations to calculate this equation properly, we must start by first calculating everything inside the parenthesis. If your answer has decimal points, round to the nearest whole number for simplicity. Here is what Bill's equation looks like once this step is finished:

$$BMR = 66 + (1{,}682) + (902) - (204)$$

Next, begin working the equation from left to right. First adding and eventually subtracting as the equation requires. Here is what the process looks like for Bill's equation:

$$BMR = 66 + (1{,}682) + (902) - (204)$$

$$BMR = 1{,}748 + (902) - (204)$$

$$BMR = 2{,}650 - (204)$$

$$BMR = 2{,}446$$

Bill's BMR is 2,446 calories. Another word, if Bill was to lie in bed for 24 hours and he doesn't move an inch, his body would burn 2,446 calories to remain functional. Keep your BMR handy because we are going to need it. Feel free to skip the next section regarding how to calculate the BMR for a woman.

Women Basal Metabolic Rate Calculation

First, let's use a hypothetical female as an example. Her name will be Jane. In order for Jane to calculate her BMR she will need to know three pieces of information. Jane will need to know her weight in pounds, height in inches, and age in years.

Jane used her bathroom scale to determine that she weighs 200 pounds.

If you don't know your height, grab a friend and a tape measure. Jane knows that she is 5 foot 5. She needs to know her height in inches. To figure this out Jane will multiply 5 times 12, since there are 12 inches in a foot, the answer Jane comes up with is 60. She then adds 5, since it is already in inches, to her previous answer of 60. Jane is 65 inches tall.

Finally, Jane knows that she is 30 years old.

Now that Jane has collected the three required pieces of information, we can finally begin to calculate Jane's BMR. The BMR calculation for women is:

$$BMR = 655 + (4.35 \times Weight\ in\ pounds)$$

$$+(4.7 \times Height\ in\ inches)$$

$$-(4.7 \times Age\ in\ years)$$

First, write out the equation and substitute the required information with your weight, height, and age. Here is what the equation looks like with Jane's information:

$$BMR = 655 + (4.35 \times 200) + (4.7 \times 65) - (4.7 \times 30)$$

Following the order of operations to calculate this equation properly, we must start by first calculating everything inside the parenthesis. If your answer has decimal points, round to the nearest whole number for simplicity. Here is what Jane's equation looks like once this is finished:

$$BMR = 655 + (870) + (306) - (141)$$

Next, begin working the equation from left to right. First adding and eventually subtracting as the equation requires. Here is what the process looks like for Jane's equation:

$$BMR = 655 + (870) + (306) - (141)$$

$$BMR = 1,525 + (306) - (141)$$

$$BMR = 1,831 - (141)$$

$$BMR = 1,690$$

Jane's BMR is 1,690 calories. Another word, if Jane was to lie in bed for 24 hours and she doesn't move an inch, her body would burn 1,690 calories to remain functional. Keep your BMR handy because you are going to need it.

Determine the Magic Number

If you recall, earlier we mentioned that in order to lose fat we need to create a calorie deficit. This means that we need to consume fewer calories than we burn in a day. Keep in mind that a healthy goal is to lose two pounds a week.

Take your BMR that you just calculated and subtract 500 from it. The reason we subtract 500 is because 500 calories a day times seven days a week equates to 3,500 calories. Since one pound of fat is equal to 3,500 calories, we will lose one pound of fat just by eating 500 calories less a day. We don't need to reduce our caloric intake any more than this because as we move and go about our daily routines, we'll actually burn more calories than our BMR. This will account for the second pound of fat that we want to lose. This new number that you calculated, your BMR minus 500 is your **magic number**. This number is how many calories you should eat in a day. If you eat this many calories a day, you will lose weight! Actually, you will likely lose a bit more than 2 pounds a week. I did. If you find this to be the case, you will need to adjust your magic number for the following week until you're only losing two pounds a week.

It isn't necessary, but I would recommend exercising if you can. It would help your efforts if you can fit a bit of cardio and weight training into your day. Recall how it is impossible to lose both fat and gain muscle at exactly the same time. Well, it is possible to lose fat one day and then gain muscle the next day which gives the appearance of doing both at the same time. The reason I recommend exercising is because there will be days when we slip and consume more than our magic number. If you are doing some cardio and weight training, that surplus of calories will go towards building muscle instead of fat. Think of exercising as your "Plan B" for those few days where our "Plan A" fails because we eat too much.

Use a bathroom scale to keep track of how much weight you lose each week. Choose a day of the week and the time of the day that you want to weigh yourself. Also, it would be best if you weighed yourself in the nude. You will get the most accurate results by always weighing yourself on the same day of the week, at the same time of day, and in the nude. Clothes will weigh differently and we tend to weigh more in the evening than we do in the morning. These are examples of how your results might become skewed. So it is important that we remain consistent.

Keeping Track

You will need to count the calories of everything you consume to ensure you stick to your magic number. This includes what you drink. It might come as a surprise that a good portion of our daily calories are consumed through beverages! Keep a simple food journal to assist you with keeping track of what you eat and how many calories those meals contain. I would recommend getting an electronic food scale. They are inexpensive and can be found just about anywhere. This will help you count the calories of foods that have serving sizes measured in grams. Counting calories is a little extra work at first, but it will be completely worth it. You will find that you tend to eat the same types of meals after a while. So all you will need to do is look at a previous time you ate that meal cutting down the time you spend on counting calories. Also, you will begin to remember how big a serving size is and how many calories it contains in the foods you like to eat. This will slowly build the habit of eating less and eating healthy. I'll use a simple turkey sandwich as an example of how to count calories.

You will be able to locate the amount of calories that a food contains either on the packaging or a quick internet search will provide the information. Below is an example of a nutrition label on a loaf of bread:

Nutrition Facts

Serving Size: 1 slice

Amount Per Serving

Calories 60	Calories from Fat 4

	% Daily Value*
Total Fat 0.5 g	1%
Saturated Fat 0 g	0%
Trans Fat 0 g	
Cholesterol 0 mg	0%
Sodium 130 mg	5%
Potassium	
Total Carbohydrate 13 g	4%
Dietary Fiber 0 g	0%
Sugars 2 g	
Sugar Alcohols	
Protein 2 g	
Vitamin A	
Vitamin C	
Calcium	
Iron	

To read the nutrition label, make note of what the serving size is. In this example, one serving size is one slice of bread. There are 60 calories in one serving. I will need two slices of bread for my turkey sandwich. Two slices of bread will equal 120 calories.

I want a slice of cheese. If I take a look at the cheese's packaging, I see that one slice of cheese contains 94 calories. Adding this to my previous total brings the calorie count to 214.

I will use one tablespoon of mayonnaise on each slice of bread. The mayonnaise jar says that one tablespoon contains 57 calories. So adding two tablespoons of mayonnaise to my previous total brings the total calories to 328.

Finally, I need to add the turkey. Two slices of turkey contain 45 calories. I decide to use four slices. Adding this to the previous total equals 418 calories. My sandwich contains 418 calories.

Below is what my food journal looks like:

Lunch:		
Turkey Sandwich		
2 slices of bread	120	
1 slice of cheese	94	
mayonnaise	114	
4 slices of turkey	90	
Total	418	

Sometimes measuring the serving size isn't as convenient as my turkey sandwich example. If the serving size is measured by weight and not easily identifiable units such as a slice of bread, then you will want to use a food scale. Eating chicken is a good example. One serving size for chicken breast is four ounces. You will want to first put the plate on the food scale and zero it out. Next, place the chicken on the plate until the food scale reads four ounces or eight ounces if you wish to eat two servings. It is a fact that most people don't have a realistic idea of what a serving size really is. Using the food scale, instead of guessing, will keep you grounded to reality. After all, when it comes to your health you don't want to guess, you want to know. Knowing allows us to evaluate our plan and make changes as needed.

Remember to record the calories you drink. Beverages will typically have a food label affixed to the container. I recommend sticking to water as much as possible. Your body actually burns more calories to heat the water to digest it, since water does not contain calories. Water is considered a negative calorie food. Negative calorie foods are foods that you burn more calories digesting it than the amount of calories they contain. Water, celery, lettuce, onions, cucumbers, and greens are all negative calorie foods. If you don't consume these foods already, consider incorporating them into your diet to help with your weight loss efforts.

You will need to count calories for your breakfast, lunch, dinner, snacks, and drinks. Let's say your magic number is 1,500 calories a day. You may want to divide this number by three, allowing yourself 500 calories for breakfast, lunch, and dinner. This will help you plan your meals. I don't believe in completely cutting certain types of food from your diet. But I think you will find that healthier food choices contain fewer calories which will allow you to eat more of it. That decision is ultimately up to you as long as you stick to your magic number.

As mentioned earlier, weigh yourself once a week. You should be losing two pounds a week. If you're not losing that much than you need to look at your food journal to see if you're eating too much. If you're losing too many pounds, you will need to increase your magic number. Weighing ourselves allows us to know what is working and what isn't and gives us the opportunity to adjust our magic number accordingly.

Reaching the Finish Line

After a while your weight loss will begin to slow. This happens because you weigh less and therefore your BMR will now be different. After a few months you will need to recalculate your magic number. Revisit the section regarding how to calculate your BMR and then subtract 500 to obtain your new magic number. It will likely be less than what it is now. This will put you back on track to losing two pounds a week.

Reaching the Finish Line

When you reach your goal weight you will want to maintain it. In order to do so, once again recalculate your magic number. You may need to actually add to it since you'll burn more calories since you will be active all day. This will take some trial and error. Continue keeping track of the amount of calories you eat and continue weighing yourself. If you are losing weight then incrementally add to your magic number until you are maintaining a steady weight. If you are losing weight then incrementally subtract from your magic number until you are maintaining a steady weight.

Conclusion

We covered a lot of information in a short amount of time! I have successfully accomplished my goal of providing you information in a short and to the point book to allow you to get started quickly on your weight loss journey today without spending weeks reading hundreds of pages. Reading and internalizing this information will mean nothing if you don't put the information to use. Implement the ideas presented in this book, and reach mastery!

Many of the diets we see advertised on television, hear friends talk about, see restaurants adjust their menus, and see food products proudly display labels such as "gluten free" are fad diets. Stay away. These don't work, at least not in the long term. They are all eventually replaced by a new fad diet. It is a vicious cycle that gets to the point where we are left confused from conflicting information and diets that don't really work.

We are all emotionally driven. Pain and pleasure are two dominate emotions that drive us to choose unhealthy eating habits. Think about situations that cause you to make unhealthy food choices, these are triggers. Now develop a plan for each trigger to help you avoid it or minimize its impact by already knowing what you will do in that situation. Your triggers and how you will mitigate your reactions should be written down in your plan.

By now you should have developed your SMART goal. A SMART goal is specific, measurable, attainable, realistic, and time-bound. Your goal should include all of these components. A SMART goal will motivate you and allow you to measure your results to let you know if you need to make adjustments.

Affirmations will help you with your weight loss goals. Your subconscious can't differentiate between the past, present, or future. Your affirmation will be emotionally charged and make use of all of your six senses as possible. By seeing yourself in your future state of weight loss, it will motivate you and your subconscious will help you make better choices. Write your affirmation down into your plan. Do your affirmation three times a day for about five minutes. Your affirmation can also be used when you are facing a difficult decision such as just staying home or going to the gym. It will likely motivate you to go to the gym.

If you didn't before, you now know that a calorie is a unit of measurement. A calorie is the amount of energy required to raise the temperature of one gram of water by one degree Celsius. One pound of fat is 3,500 calories. In order to lose weight you need to create a deficit of calories. To lose fat you need to create a calorie deficit, to gain muscle (or fat) you need a surplus of calories. It is a physiological impossibility to lose fat and gain muscle at the exact same time. By consuming fewer calories, your body will burn fat to compensate which will cause you to lose weight.

To create this deficit, you need to calculate your magic number using the BMR calculation specific to your sex and then subtracting 500. The magic number is the amount of calories you need to consume every day. You will know how many calories you consume by counting them in the foods you eat. You will need to weight yourself every week and make minor adjustments to your magic number as necessary. After a few months you will weigh less and need to recalculate your magic number.

Once you reach your goal weight, recalculate your BMR and this time you will likely need to add to it, not subtract like before. Continue weighing yourself and make adjustments as necessary. You may need to add calories or consume fewer calories to maintain your weight.

I want to personally commend you for making the decision to improve your health. I can't even begin to express the joy I felt once I finally met my target weight. This is an amazing joy that you will get to experience.

Below is my real weight loss plan when I started. I've included it so that you may use it as an example in preparing your plan and the strategies you will use on your weight loss journey.

My plan:

Starting weight: 317 lbs

Triggers:
* Annoyed by co-workers so I drive to McDonalds as a reason to get out of the office
* Overeat because of childhood habit of not getting meals
* Multiple fast food restaurants on my drive home from work

Responses to triggers:
* Go for a walk at lunch to get a break from co-workers
* Keep a large amount of food in the house
* ~~Take~~ Take the by-pass highway home instead so I'm not tempted

Goal:
To lose 67 pounds of fat and weigh 250 by December 8, 2012.
* weigh yourself every Saturday morning when I wake up.

Affirmation:
I have a slender physic with firm fitting clothes. I walk into a restaurant or store and I notice women stop what they are doing & look at me and check me out!

Magic number:
BMR= 2,731.81 - 500 = 2,231 calories per day

My food journal, Day 1:

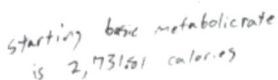

starting basic metabolic rate
is 2,731561 calories

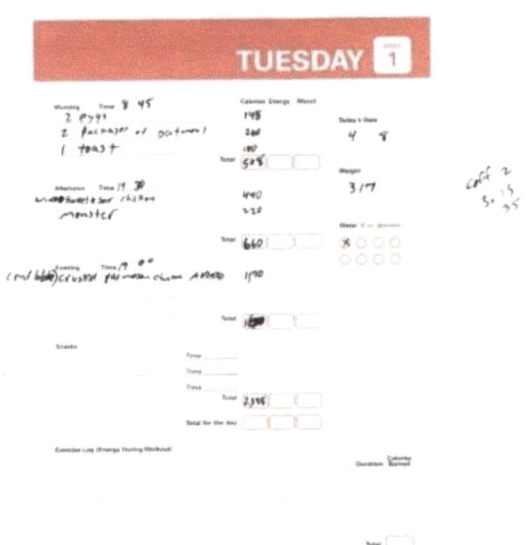

My food journal, Day 2:

WEDNESDAY 1

Morning   Time 09 00
Breakfast coffee 111   milk 110   356
2 packages of oatmeal   260
2 eggs   144
                                    Total: 744

Today's Diary
4 9

Weight
319

Afternoon Time 12 00
baked chicken   110
mixed vegas   60
A 2 Sauce   25
                                    Total: 195

Evening   Time 17 30
oatmeal 2   200
Pierogies 2 serv.   440
string beans   60
                                    Total: 700

Snacks
Apple w/peanut butter   Time 14 46 350
mixed food   Time 19 30 160
                         Time
                                    Total: 490

Total for the day 2249

Exercise Log (Energy During Workout)

Calories
Duration   Burned

Total:

6

A sample of tracking my weight using Excel:

Date	Weight	Notes
April 8, 2014	317	Starting weight
April 12, 2014	314	
April 19, 2014	312	

www.ingramcontent.com/pod-product-compliance
Lightning Source LLC
Chambersburg PA
CBHW050834290526
45792CB00001B/389